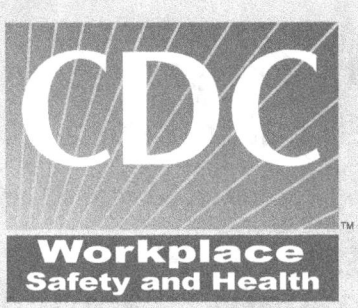

I0426402

Evaluation of Antimony and Mercury Exposure in Fire Fighters

Marie A. de Perio, MD

Srinivas Durgam, MSPH, MSChE, CIH

Health Hazard Evaluation Report
HETA 2009-0025 and HETA 2009-0076-3085
Boca Raton Fire Rescue Services
Boca Raton, Florida
Tamarac Fire Rescue
Tamarac, Florida
June 2009

DEPARTMENT OF HEALTH AND HUMAN SERVICES
Centers for Disease Control and Prevention

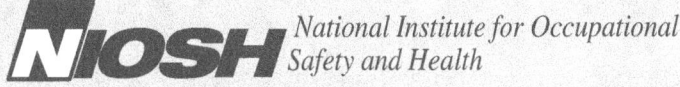

National Institute for Occupational Safety and Health

The employer shall post a copy of this report for a period of 30 calendar days at or near the workplace(s) of affected employees. The employer shall take steps to insure that the posted determinations are not altered, defaced, or covered by other material during such period. [37 FR 23640, November 7, 1972, as amended at 45 FR 2653, January 14, 1980].

CONTENTS

ABBREVIATIONS

ACGIH®	American Conference of Governmental Industrial Hygienists
AMA	American Medical Association
ATSDR	Agency for Toxic Substances and Disease Registry
BRFRS	Boca Raton Fire Rescue Services
CDC	Centers for Disease Control and Prevention
FFR®	Fibrous flame retardant
HHE	Health hazard evaluation
IAFF	International Association of Fire Fighters
LOD	Limit of detection
µg/g	Micrograms per gram
µg/L	Micrograms per liter
NAICS	North American Industry Classification System
NFPA	National Fire Protection Association
NIOSH	National Institute for Occupational Safety and Health
TFR	Tamarac Fire Rescue

The National Institute for Occupational Safety and Health (NIOSH) conducted health hazard evaluations (HHEs) at Boca Raton Fire Rescue Services (BRFRS) in Boca Raton, Florida and at Tamarac Rescue Services (TFR) in Tamarac, Florida. The HHEs concerned potential exposure of fire fighters to antimony from wearing pants made from FireWear® fabric. Site visits were made February 2–6, 2009.

What NIOSH Did

- We reviewed hair and urine test results performed by BRFRS fire fighters' personal physicians.

- We administered to 66 participants questionnaires about personal characteristics and work history.

- We collected urine samples and measured urine antimony and mercury levels.

What NIOSH Found

- Fire fighters from BRFRS and TFR had urine antimony levels that were below or within the expected range for the general population. This was true whether or not they had been wearing pants made from FireWear fabric.

- Wearing pants made from FireWear fabric did not pose a health hazard from antimony exposure.

- Fire fighters from BRFRS and TFR had urine mercury levels that were below or within the expected range for the general population.

What Fire Executive Staff Can Do

- Continue to issue station uniforms that comply with the National Fire Protection Association (NFPA) 1975 standard. The pants made from FireWear fabric are one type of uniform pants that meet this standard.

- Facilitate the evaluation of fire fighters with work-related health concerns by a residency-trained and/or board-certified occupational medicine specialist or medical toxicologist.

What Fire Fighters Can Do

- Continue to wear station uniforms that comply with the NFPA 1975 standard.

- Follow garment label instructions when washing station uniforms.

- Notify the battalion chief or other chief officers about possible work-related health concerns.

- Seek medical care for work-related health concerns from a residency-trained and/or board-certified occupational medicine specialist or medical toxicologist.

- Evaluate the quality of the health information found on the Internet. Ensure that information is reliable, up-to-date, and unbiased.

This page intentionally left blank

SUMMARY

NIOSH investigators evaluated fire fighters' exposure to antimony. Wearing pants made of FireWear fabric did not cause elevated levels of antimony among fire fighters or pose a health hazard from antimony exposure to those who wore them. We recommend continued use of station uniforms that comply with the NFPA 1975 standard.

In October 2008, NIOSH received an HHE request from the Fire Chief at BRFRS in Boca Raton, Florida. The request concerned the possible exposure of BRFRS fire fighters to antimony through their station uniform pants made of FireWear® fabric. FireWear fabric contains antimony trioxide, which is often used for its flame retardant properties. In the weeks before the HHE request, 30 fire fighters had undergone hair testing for heavy metals after one fire fighter reported unexplained symptoms. All fire fighters were reported by the laboratory to have elevated antimony levels in their hair samples. As a result, BRFRS fire fighters ceased wearing the pants department-wide prior to submitting in early October 2008, and the HHE request was submitted.

NIOSH investigators contacted the Acting Fire Chief at TFR in Tamarac, Florida to seek TFR participation in the HHE because its fire fighters were wearing uniform pants made from the FireWear fabric. In January 2009, NIOSH received an HHE request from the Acting TFR Fire Chief to evaluate antimony exposure in TFR fire fighters.

We reviewed laboratory results for 30 BRFRS fire fighters who had submitted workers' compensation claims. Hair testing results for the 30 fire fighters, all from the same commercial laboratory, were reported as elevated. Twenty-three of these 30 fire fighters also underwent urine heavy metal testing by the same commercial laboratory. Only one fire fighter was found to have an elevated urine antimony level, but all 23 fire fighters had mercury levels that exceeded the testing laboratory's reference range. Though the laboratory reports stated that these were urine samples collected without any provocation, during our site visit some fire fighters verbally reported receiving a provoking agent prior to urine collection.

During our on-site evaluation at BRFRS and TFR in February 2009, we met with fire executive staff and union representatives. We also administered questionnaires to participants that included personal characteristics, work history, and possible sources of exposure to antimony and mercury. We collected urine samples, which were analyzed for antimony and mercury by the National Center for Environmental Health at CDC.

Twenty BRFRS fire fighters and 42 TFR fire fighters participated. All TFR participants had worn pants made from FireWear fabric while on duty in the preceding 2 weeks, and they reported wearing these pants for an average of 92 hours, or close to four 24-hour shifts, during this time.

All BRFRS participants and all but one TFR participant were found to have urine antimony levels below or within the laboratory reference range for the general population. One TFR participant had a urine antimony level just above the upper limit of the laboratory reference range.

Urine antimony levels of BRFRS and TFR participants were not significantly different. No BRFRS or TFR participant had a urine mercury level higher than the laboratory reference range. Urine mercury levels of BRFRS and TFR participants were not significantly different.

Wearing pants made from FireWear fabric did not pose a health hazard from antimony exposure. Reliable and recommended testing methods with well-validated reference ranges should be used to measure the concentration of heavy metals in the body when health symptoms are consistent with overexposure to these metals. We recommend continued use of station uniforms that comply with the NFPA 1975 standard. Pants made from FireWear fabric are one product that meets this standard.

Keywords: NAICS 922160 (Fire Protection), fire fighter, antimony, mercury, uniforms, urine testing

INTRODUCTION

On October 24, 2008, NIOSH received an HHE request from the Fire Chief of BRFRS regarding antimony exposure among fire fighters. The concern began with one fire fighter who had been experiencing unexplained neurologic symptoms, including hoarseness, weakness, and numbness, since October 2007. He had seen multiple physicians, but no diagnosis was made. In July 2008, the fire fighter sought the care of a holistic medicine physician who performed heavy metals testing on a hair sample through a commercial laboratory. This test revealed an elevated level of antimony.

Subsequent to this finding, the Boca Raton IAFF, Local 1560 encouraged all 199 Boca Raton fire fighters to undergo testing for antimony. As of November 15, 2008, 44 workers' compensation claims had been submitted by fire fighters claiming exposure to antimony. Although many of the claimants did not report any adverse health effects, those who did reported headaches, fatigue, and joint and muscle pain. Thirty of these fire fighters underwent hair testing for heavy metals at the same laboratory as the initial fire fighter. All were reported by the laboratory to have elevated antimony levels in their hair samples. Mercury levels in hair and urine samples were also reported to be high among the fire fighters.

Some fire fighters at BRFRS hypothesized that they had been exposed to antimony through their station uniform pants, which contain antimony trioxide for its flame retardant properties. The fire department recalled the pants from fire fighters in early October 2008 as a result of these concerns.

Fire fighter station uniforms made from FireWear fabric (Spring Industries, Incorporated, Fort Mill, South Carolina) consist of 55% FFR fiber and 45% cotton. The FFR fiber is a patented, engineered modacrylic, consisting of the Protex® fiber (Kaneka Corporation, Osaka, Japan), which contains acrylonitrile, vinylidene chloride, and antimony trioxide. Upon exposure to temperatures reaching 450–500°F, antimony and chlorine components within the fiber vaporize to form three gases: antimony chloride, antimony oxychloride, and hydrogen chloride. These gases are all flame retardants and work to extinguish a fire by quenching free radicals, diluting flammable gases near the fabric surface, and shielding oxygen from feeding the flame front. FireWear fabric does not drip, melt, or separate. Station uniforms made from FireWear fabric meet the requirements set by the NFPA 1975: Standard on Station/Work Uniforms for Emergency Services [NFPA 2009]. Fire departments across the country, including departments in Boston, Chicago, and Charleston, wear uniform pants made from the FireWear fabric.

Media reports and fire fighter online blogs caused national concern over the safety of uniform pants containing antimony. Fire fighters in fire departments across the country and members of the IAFF and its local organizations expressed concern, and multiple fire departments discontinued use of these pants. NIOSH investigators contacted the Acting Fire Chief at TFR in Tamarac, Florida to seek its participation because at that time its fire fighters were wearing uniform pants made from FireWear fabric. On January 23, 2009, NIOSH received an HHE request from the Acting Fire Chief at TFR to evaluate antimony exposure in TFR fire fighters. Two weeks before submitting the request, TFR fire executive staff issued a policy allowing individual fire fighters to decide whether or not to continue use of these pants.

Antimony

Antimony is a silver-white metal that is found in the earth's crust. It is found at very low levels throughout the environment. According to ATSDR, most of the general population in the United States is exposed to low levels of antimony every day, primarily in food, drinking water, and air [ATSDR 1992]. ATSDR is an agency within the Department of Health and Human Services. Antimony is used in the production of ceramics, glass, paints, pigments, fireworks, alloys, batteries, and semiconductors. Antimony compounds, particularly antimony oxides, are also used as flame retardants in textiles, plastics, rubber, adhesives, and paper [Stokinger 1981; Carson et al. 1986; Winship 1987].

Signs and symptoms of acute exposure to antimony include abdominal pain, cough, loss of appetite, itching, and irritation of the skin, eyes, nose, and throat. Signs and symptoms of chronic exposure include headache, sleeplessness, dizziness, metallic taste, weight loss, nausea, vomiting, diarrhea, impairment of sense of smell, and pain or tightness in the chest [NIOSH 1988]. Neurological effects have not been observed in humans following inhalation, oral, or intravenous exposure to antimony [ATSDR 1992]. No studies have been published about the health effects in humans following dermal exposure to antimony or about dermal absorption of antimony in humans or animals [ATSDR 1992]. Antimony trioxide has been characterized as "possibly carcinogenic" to humans by the International Agency for Research on Cancer [IARC 1989]. This means that there is inadequate evidence in humans and limited evidence in experimental animals to suggest carcinogenicity.

Urine testing is the recommended method of testing for antimony [Goldfrank et al. 2006]. Hair sampling is not validated, it is not recommended by the AMA or the ATSDR for heavy metals, and its results are unreliable [AMA 1994; ATSDR 2001]. The laboratory reference range is the range of levels expected in the general population for antimony. The reference range in urine is 0.130–0.340 μg/L or 0.120–0.364 μg/g creatinine [CDC 2005]. Creatinine is a waste product that is excreted from the body by the kidneys, and it can be used as a marker for urine dilution. The laboratory reference range is based on data from 2,690 individuals, a representative sample of the civilian, non-institutionalized population in the United States [CDC 2005]. The geometric mean urine antimony concentration for the general population is 0.134 μg/L or 0.126 μg/g creatinine [CDC 2005]. The half-life of antimony in urine is approximately 95 hours [Kentner et al. 1995].

A previous study, published by Edelman and colleagues, found that urine antimony levels of fire fighters responding to the World Trade Center fires and collapse were significantly higher than those of New York City fire fighters who were assigned to office duties as a result of prior injury [Edelman et al. 2003]. However, levels among World Trade Center responders were still within the reference range found in the general population [CDC 2005]. One hypothesis for this difference was that the World Trade Center fire fighters were exposed to antimony as a byproduct of combustion. When upholstery or other fabric made with antimony-containing fire retardant fibers burns, the ashes remaining may be aerosolized and inhaled if respiratory protection is not maintained throughout the cleanup stages of the fire. These fire fighters were wearing no clothing or gear containing antimony compounds, so their exposures would have been through products of combustion, smoking, or through normal environmental exposures. To our knowledge, this is the only published study concerning the exposure of fire fighters to antimony.

Mercury

Mercury is a naturally occurring metal found in air, water, and soil. It exists in several forms including elemental, inorganic compounds, and organic compounds. The general population is primarily exposed to elemental mercury vapor from dental amalgam and to organic mercury from dietary sources such as fish. Occupational exposure to mercury can occur in dentistry, mining, and the manufacture of electrical equipment and medical instruments [Evans 1998]. Accumulated mercury in the ecosystem is known to be released during wildfires in forests, which may present an additional route of exposure to fire fighters [Weidinmyer and Friedly 2007]. The study by Edelman and colleagues did not find urine mercury levels of World Trade Center fire fighters to be different from those of fire fighters not present at the World Trade Center disaster [Edelman et al. 2003]. To our knowledge, no other studies looking at urine mercury levels among fire fighters have been published.

Signs of mercury toxicity vary with the form of mercury and the route of exposure and can include gingivitis, mouth sores, and excessive salivation. These signs typically occur with urine levels greater than 300 µg/L [Magos and Clarkson 2006]. Neurologic effects can include personality changes, irritability, fatigue, tremor, ataxia, memory and concentration deficits, sleep disturbances, and a metallic taste. Mercury toxicity can also lead to kidney damage [Brodkin et al. 2007].

Although many laboratories indicate that only urine levels above 150 µg/g of creatinine should be considered toxic, evidence suggests that early signs of mercury intoxication can be seen in workers excreting more than 50 µg/g of creatinine [Barregard et al. 1988; Echeverria et al. 1995]. ACGIH currently recommends that inorganic mercury in workers' urine not exceed 35 µg/g of creatinine [ACGIH 2009].

Urine and blood are the recommended sources for measuring inorganic mercury in the body [Goldfrank et al. 2006]. The laboratory reference range for mercury in urine is 0 580–3.99 µg/L or 0.650–3.00 µg/g creatinine. This reference range is based on data from 1,960 individuals from a representative sample [CDC 2005]. The geometric mean urine mercury concentration for the general population is 0.606 µg/L, or 0.620 µg/g creatinine [CDC 2005]. The half-life of mercury in the urine is approximately 1–3 months [Roels et al. 1991; Jonsson et al. 1999].

Review of Workers' Compensation Records

On November 13, 2009, we requested the workers' compensation claims submitted in the preceding 2 months from the city of Boca Raton.

Measurement of Urine Antimony and Mercury Levels

On February 2–6, 2009, we conducted a site visit to BRFRS and TFR. We met with fire executive staff, union leaders, and city officials during the opening conference at each department. Also present at the opening conference at BRFRS was an attorney from a law firm representing a group of BRFRS fire fighters. We invited 112 employees at BRFRS to participate, including 42 on-duty fire fighters, 50 additional fire fighters who had submitted workers' compensation claims, and 20 chief officers and fire inspectors. None of the participating BRFRS employees had since October 2008 worn pants made from FireWear fabric. We invited 96 TFR employees to be screened for participation, including 70 on-duty fire fighters, 16 off-duty fire fighters, and 10 chief officers and fire inspectors. The TFR employees who had worn FireWear pants while on duty in the previous 2 weeks were eligible to participate. A 2-week cutoff was chosen because this period represents the time at which very little antimony is expected to remain in the body based on the known rate of removal.

Employees were informed of the HHEs by both fire executive staff and NIOSH investigators. We explained the objectives and methods of our evaluation to all of the on-duty BRFRS fire fighters and most of the on-duty TFR fire fighters, answered their questions, and disseminated written information on antimony, mercury, and hair testing. After obtaining informed consent, we administered questionnaires to participants that included questions concerning personal characteristics, work history, and possible sources of exposure to antimony and mercury. For our job title classification, the fire fighter category included fire fighters, fire fighter-drivers, and fire fighter-paramedics. Company officers included lieutenants and captains, while chief officers included battalion, assistant, division, and fire chiefs. We also offered confidential interviews to employees with health and workplace concerns. Two participants requested confidential interviews.

We collected one-time urine samples to measure antimony and mercury. These urine samples were shipped on dry ice to the Inorganic Toxicology Laboratory in the Division of Laboratory Sciences at the National Center for Environmental Health at CDC in Atlanta, Georgia, on February 5 and 6, 2009.

Urine levels of antimony and mercury were measured by inductively coupled dynamic reaction cell plasma mass spectrometry following published protocols [Caldwell et al. 2005]. Urine specimens were analyzed for creatinine using a commercial enzymatic kit (Roche Diagnostics, Indianapolis, Indiana). The laboratory results were reviewed and approved by a quality assurance officer to ensure that they conformed to acceptable quality standards. The antimony and mercury levels were then adjusted for urine creatinine.

The analytical LOD is the level at which the measurement of a chemical has a 95% probability of being greater than zero [Taylor 1987]. The analytical LOD for antimony was 0.032 µg/L, while the analytical LOD for mercury was 0.08 µg/L.

Statistical Analysis

Statistical analysis was performed using SAS 9.2 (SAS Institute, Cary, North Carolina). We calculated the geometric mean urine antimony and mercury levels for both BRFRS and TFR participants. Concentrations less than the LOD were assigned a value equal to the LOD divided by the square root of 2 [Taylor 1987]. Because urine antimony and mercury levels were log normally distributed among participants, we compared the means of the log transformed values for urine antimony and mercury levels between participant groups using the Student's t-test. We also calculated means and proportions of variables from the questionnaire.

Review of Workers' Compensation Records

We reviewed 44 claims that had been submitted to the City of Boca Raton by November 15, 2008. Claims for 30 fire fighters contained laboratory results. All hair testing results were from the same commercial laboratory and were reported as elevated, though two different reference ranges were used. Twenty-three of the 30 fire fighters who underwent hair testing also underwent urine testing by the same laboratory. One of these 23 fire fighters was found to have an elevated urine antimony level of 1.2 µg/g creatinine compared to the given laboratory reference range of <0.6 µg/g creatinine. We calculated the geometric mean urine antimony concentration for these 23 fire fighters to be 0.23 µg/g creatinine, with a range of 0.1–1.2 µg/g creatinine. We also noted that all 23 fire fighters who had urine heavy metal testing had mercury levels higher than the given laboratory reference range of 3 µg/g creatinine. The geometric mean urine mercury concentration of these 23 fire fighters was 13.75 µg/g creatinine, with a range of 4.2–40 µg/g creatinine. Though the laboratory reports stated that these were urine samples collected without any provocation, during our site visit some fire fighters reported they had been administered a provoking agent prior to urine collection.

Questionnaire Results

Twenty of 112 invited BRFRS fire fighters took part. These participants included 2 fire fighters, 3 company officers, 3 fire inspectors, and 12 chief officers. Also participating were 4 civilian employees who were not fire fighters, giving a total of 24 BRFRS participants. Demographic and work characteristics of BRFRS participants are shown in Tables 1 and 2.

Of the 96 invited TFR fire fighters, 42 were eligible to participate because they had worn pants made from FireWear fabric in the previous 2 weeks. All 42 participated. The participants included 29 fire fighters, 9 company officers, 2 fire inspectors, and 2 chief officers. Demographic and work characteristics of TFR participants are shown in Tables 1 and 2.

TFR participants wore FireWear pants for a mean of 92 hours, or close to four 24-hour shifts, during the previous 2 weeks. TFR participants reported wearing the FireWear pants for 4 years and owned four pairs of the pants, on average.

Table 1. Demographic characteristics of participants

Demographic characteristic	BRFRS (n=24) No. (%)	TFR (n=42) No. (%)
Age (mean)	49.3 years	39.0 years
Male sex	23 (95.8%)	39 (92.9%)
Race		
White	21 (87.5%)	39 (92.9%)
Asian	1 (4.2%)	1 (2.4%)
African American	2 (8.3%)	0 (0%)
American Indian	0 (0%)	1 (2.4%)
Bi-racial	0 (0%)	1 (2.4%)
Hispanic ethnicity	2 (8.3%)	10 (23.8%)
Current smoker	2 (8.3%)	1 (2.4%)

Table 2. Work characteristics of participants

Work characteristic	BRFRS (n=24) No. (%)	TFR (n=42) No. (%)
Job title		
Fire fighter	2 (8.3%)	29 (69.0%)
Company officer	3 (12.5%)	9 (21.4%)
Inspector	3 (12.5%)	2 (4.8%)
Chief officer	12 (50.0%)	2 (4.8%)
Civilian employee	4 (16.7%)	0 (0%)
Years as fire fighter (mean)	25.8 years	12.7 years
Years at BRFRS/TFR (mean)	22.8 years	10.9 years

Urine Antimony Measurements

The geometric mean urine antimony levels of BRFRS and TFR participants are shown in Figure 1.

Four BRFRS participants and nine TFR participants were found to have urine antimony levels below the analytical LOD of 0.032 µg/L. All BRFRS participants and all but one TFR participant were found to have creatinine-corrected urine antimony levels below or within the laboratory reference range of 0.120–0.364 µg/g creatinine for the general population [CDC 2005]. One TFR participant had a urine antimony level of 0.366 µg/g creatinine, a negligible difference from the upper limit of the laboratory reference range. The range of urine antimony levels for BRFRS participants was 0.027–0.285 µg/g creatinine, while the range of urine antimony levels for TFR participants was 0.017–0.366 µg/g creatinine.

The geometric mean urine antimony level was 0.063 µg/g creatinine for BRFRS participants, 0.054 µg/g creatinine for TFR participants, and 0.126 µg/g creatinine for the general population (shown in Figure 3) [CDC 2005]. The means of the log transformed urine antimony levels of BRFRS and TFR participants were not significantly different (p=0.31). However, the mean of the log transformed urine antimony levels of BRFRS and TFR participants was significantly lower than that of the general population (p<0.001). Only two BRFRS (8.3%) participants and four TFR (9 5%) participants had urine antimony levels higher than the geometric mean for the general population.

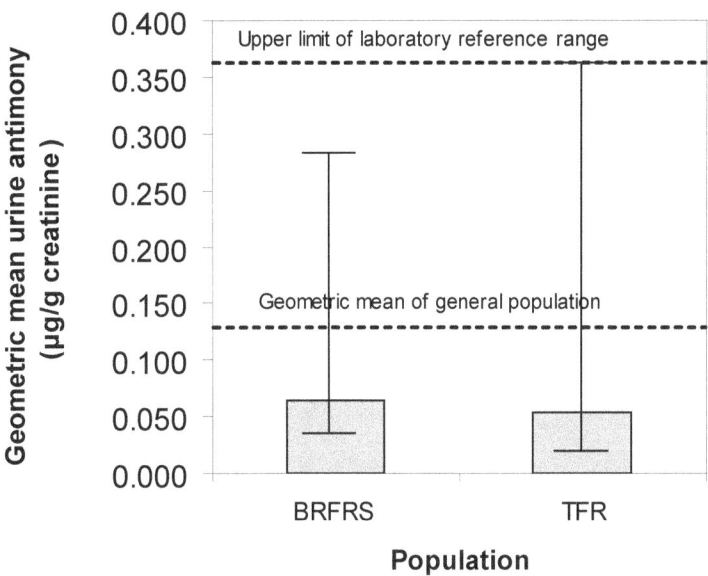

Figure 1. Geometric mean urine antimony levels of BRFRS and TFR fire fighters

Urine antimony levels were similar among the 62 fire service employees and the 4 civilian employees. Urine antimony levels were also similar between a group comprised of fire fighters and company officers and another group comprised of inspectors and chief officers.

None of the participants from either fire department reported participating in other work activities that might expose them to antimony, including metal smelting or battery, ceramics, and flame-retardant materials manufacturing. None of the participants reported being treated with pentavalent antimony, also known as sodium stibogluconate or Pentostam™ for any parasitic diseases in the previous 2 weeks.

Four participants who reported shooting firearms in the previous 2 weeks had urine antimony levels that were similar to the levels of those who did not shoot firearms. Urine antimony levels were also similar among the three participants who were current smokers and those who were non-smokers.

Urine Mercury Measurements

The geometric mean urine mercury levels of BRFRS and TFR participants are shown in Figure 2.

No BRFRS or TFR participants were found to have a creatinine-corrected urine mercury level higher than the laboratory reference range of 0.650–3.00 µg/g creatinine [CDC 2005]. The range of urine mercury levels for BRFRS participants was 0.143–1.013 µg/g creatinine, while the range of urine mercury levels for TFR participants was 0.220–2.810 µg/g creatinine.

The means of the log transformed values for urine mercury levels of BRFRS and TFR participants were not significantly different (p= 0.62). The geometric mean urine mercury level was 0.805 µg/g creatinine for BRFRS participants, 0.734 µg/g creatinine for TFR participants, and 0.620 µg/g creatinine for the general population (shown in Figure 4) [CDC 2005]. Fifteen BRFRS (62.5%) and 26 TFR (61.9%) participants had urine mercury levels that were higher than the geometric mean for the general population. However, the means of the log transformed mercury levels of BRFRS and TFR participants and the general population were not significantly different (p=0.12).

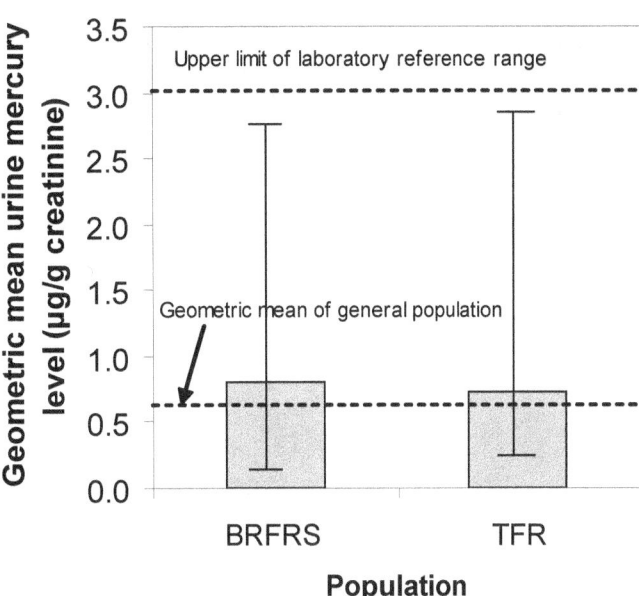

Figure 2. Geometric mean urine mercury levels of BRFRS and TFR fire fighters

None of the participants from either fire department reported participating in other work activities that might expose them to mercury, including chloralkali production and thermometer manufacturing.

Each participant was informed in writing of his or her individual urine test results and their significance within 4 weeks after urine collection.

DISCUSSION

We found that fire fighters from BRFRS and TFR had urine antimony levels that fell below or within the normal range for the general population whether or not the fire fighters were wearing pants made from FireWear fabric. Our results indicate that wearing these pants did not pose a risk for antimony toxicity. It does not appear that fire fighters at these fire departments were exposed to high levels of antimony during the course of their work. Furthermore, we found that, on average, fire fighters from both departments had urine antimony levels that fell below the average level for the general population. Possible reasons for this difference include regional differences in the amount of antimony present in food and drinking water and random variation that can be found when comparing a small group to a large group.

DISCUSSION

Only 17 9% of invited BRFRS fire fighters participated in our HHE, compared to 100% of eligible TFR fire fighters. It is likely that two factors played a role in the low participation at BRFRS. First, the law firm representing a group of BRFRS fire fighters advised its clients not to participate in our HHE. This advice also likely influenced those fire fighters who were not part of pending litigation in their decision not to participate. At the request of the law firm representing BRFRS fire fighters, we shared copies of our HHE protocol, informed consent document, and questionnaire during our site visit. Second, many of the fire fighters who had already had hair testing done reported receiving medical advice from their personal physician that urine testing for heavy metals was inferior to hair testing. During our site visit, several BRFRS fire fighters informed us that they had found information on the Internet that supported this medical advice. It is unclear whether the low participation rate at BRFRS influenced the results.

Urine testing is the most reliable and valid test method for measuring antimony levels in the body [Goldfrank et al. 2006]. Along with blood testing, urine sampling is also a preferred method for measuring mercury levels in the body. CDC has established reference ranges for urine levels of antimony and mercury for the general population [CDC 2005]. This evaluation highlights the importance of using validated laboratory methods in screening, diagnosing, and treating employees.

Hair testing is not a reliable or valid method for measuring levels of heavy metals in the body, except for methylmercury [Harkins and Susten 2003]. It has many limitations. First, accepted standards on methods of collection, storage, and analysis of hair are lacking. Second, problems exist with the regulation and certification of laboratories conducting hair analysis. It has been shown that different laboratories can report different results for hair samples collected from the same person and can report different reference ranges [Seidel et al. 2001]. Third, CDC has not established reference ranges for hair levels of antimony and mercury for the general population. Fourth, hair analysis cannot distinguish between internal exposure (substances inside one's body) and external exposure (substances that might stick to the hair, like those in hair care products or antimony-containing ash from fires). Fifth, hair analysis for heavy metals does not predict toxicity or disease [Harkins and Susten 2003].

The AMA current policy on hair testing reads: "The AMA opposes chemical analysis of the hair as a determinant of the need for medical therapy and supports informing the American public and appropriate governmental agencies of this unproven practice and its potential for healthcare fraud" [AMA 1994].

Furthermore, in 2001, the ATSDR convened a seven-member panel in Atlanta, Georgia, to review and discuss the current state of the science related to hair analysis in assessing environmental exposures. This panel concluded that: "For most substances, insufficient data currently exist that would allow the prediction of a health effect from the concentration of the substance in hair. The presence of a substance in hair may indicate exposure (both internal and external), but does not necessarily indicate the source of exposure" [ATSDR 2001].

Testing of the pants for antimony compounds was not conducted as part of this evaluation. If antimony were being released from the pants and absorbed through the skin, the urine tests would have indicated that fire fighters wearing pants made from FireWear fabric had levels higher than (1) the U.S. population and (2) the fire fighters not wearing these pants. We found no differences between these groups. Also, a private technical consulting and engineering firm previously tested the Protex fiber, which is found in FireWear fabric. The firm's researchers concluded that antimony trioxide exposures associated with use of clothing made from these fibers comply with the standards under California's Safe Drinking Water and Toxic Enforcement Act of 1986 (Proposition 65) [Geomatrix Consultants 2006].

We found that urine mercury levels for all participating fire fighters were similar to those of the general population. Elevated urine mercury levels in the 23 BRFRS fire fighters that submitted workers' compensation claims could have been artificially raised by the administration of a chelating agent. Though the laboratory reports stated that these were urine samples collected without any provocation, during our site visit, some fire fighters reported they had been administered a chelating agent prior to urine collection. Chelating agents act as scavengers by collecting small amounts of metals such as mercury and antimony from the body and forcing them to be excreted. This creates an artificial and temporary increase in urine mercury levels. Because laboratory reference ranges are representative of a healthy population under non-challenge or non-provoked conditions, interpretation of provoked urine results is difficult. In this case, the commercial laboratory that analyzed mercury levels in urine specimens of the 23 BRFRS fire fighters compared the results to a reference range based on a non-challenged collection. Results from post-chelation-challenge urine tests do not provide sufficient evidence of metal toxicity. Contamination during the collection, processing, and analysis of the samples could have also caused an artificial increase in urine mercury levels.

CONCLUSIONS

Wearing pants made from FireWear fabric did not pose a health hazard from antimony exposure. Fire fighters from BRFRS and TFR had urine antimony levels that fell below or within the normal range for the general population whether or not the fire fighters were wearing pants that contain antimony trioxide.

RECOMMENDATIONS

Based on our findings, we recommend the actions listed below to promote the health and safety of fire fighters.

1. BRFRS and TFR should continue to issue, and its fire fighters should continue to wear, station uniforms that comply with the NFPA 1975: Standard on Station/Work Uniforms for Emergency Services [NFPA 2009]. Pants made from FireWear fabric are one product that meets this standard.

2. Fire fighters should follow garment label instructions when laundering station uniforms. Labels on garments made from FireWear fabric suggesting low temperature washing and laundering without chlorine bleach are consistent with instructions for fabrics containing cotton and FFR fibers. These instructions are designed to ensure that the garment remains durable and does not lose color; they do not address the release of antimony.

3. Fire fighters should notify their battalion chief or other chief officers about any possible work-related health problems.

4. Fire fighters should seek medical care from qualified medical professionals for any health concerns. Fire fighters should ensure that their physicians are certified by appropriate medical specialty boards by checking the American Board of Medical Specialties website at www.abms.org/. Fire fighters

should also ensure that their physicians possess a current medical license from the state medical board by checking the Florida Department of Health's license verification website at ww2.doh.state.fl.us/IRM00PRAES/PRASLIST ASP. This website also lists any disciplinary action taken against each physician. Fire fighters should also seek medical care for work-related health concerns from a residency-trained and/or board-certified occupational medicine specialist or medical toxicologist. The American College of Occupational and Environmental Medicine website at www.acoem.org/ and the American College of Medical Toxicologists website at www.acmt.net/findtoxicologist.html list appropriate medical providers. It may be helpful for fire executive staff to locate an appropriate physician for the department and facilitate contact.

5. The decision to perform laboratory testing for heavy metals, including antimony and mercury, should be based on whether or not documented health symptoms are consistent with overexposure to these metals. It is important to use reliable and recommended testing methods with well-validated reference ranges to measure the concentration of heavy metals in the body. Because results from elemental hair analysis and post-chelation-challenge urine tests do not provide sufficient evidence of heavy metal toxicity, they should not be used to justify searching the workplace for exposures or to treat heavy metal toxicity. In particular, they should not be used to justify chelation therapy, which can be potentially harmful to a patient.

6. Given the abundance of information available on the Internet, fire fighters should evaluate the quality of the health information that they find. It is important to ensure that health information is reliable, up-to-date, and unbiased. The National Library of Medicine and the National Institutes of Health offer guidelines for evaluating the quality of health information on the Internet on their website at www.nlm.nih.gov/medlineplus/evaluatinghealthinformation.html.

REFERENCES

ACGIH [2009]. 2009 TLVs® and BEIs®: threshold limit values for chemical substances and physical agents and biological exposure indices. Cincinnati, OH: American Conference of Governmental Industrial Hygienists.

AMA [1994]. Hair analysis: a potential for abuse. Policy No. H-175.995. Chicago, IL: American Medical Association. Reaffirmed 2004.

ATSDR [1992]. Toxicological profile for antimony. Atlanta, GA: U.S. Department of Health and Human Services, Agency for Toxic Substances and Disease Registry.

ATSDR [2001]. Hair analysis panel discussion: exploring the state of the science. Summary Report. Atlanta, GA: U.S. Department of Health and Human Services, Agency for Toxic Substances and Disease Registry [http://www atsdr.cdc. gov/hac/hair_analysis/index.html]. Date accessed: March 2009.

Barregard L, Hultberg B, Schutz A, Sallsten G [1998]. Enzymuria in workers exposed to inorganic mercury. Int Arch Occup Environ Hlth 61:65–69.

Brodkin E, Copes R, Mattman A, Kennedy J, Kling R, Yassi A [2007]. Lead and mercury exposures: interpretation and action. CMAJ 176:59–63.

Caldwell K, Hartel J, Jarrett J, Jones RL [2005]. Inductively coupled plasma mass spectrometry to measure multiple toxic elements in urine in NHANES 1999-2000. Atomic Spectroscopy 26:1–7.

Carson BL, Ellis HV, McCann JL [1986]. Antimony. In: Toxicology and biological monitoring of metal in humans. Chelsea, MI: Lewis, pp. 21–26.

CDC [2005]. Third national report on human exposure to environmental chemicals. Atlanta, GA: U.S. Department of Health and Human Services, Centers for Disease Control and Prevention.

Echeverria D, Heyer NJ, Martin MD, Naleway CA, Woods JS, Bittner AC [1995]. Behavioral effects of low-level exposure to Hg among dentists. Neurotoxicol Teratol 17:161–168.

Edelman P, Osterloh J, Pirkle J, Caudill S, Grainger J, Jones R, Blount B, Calafat A, Turner W, Feldman D, Baron S, Bernard B,

REFERENCES
(CONTINUED)

Lushniak B, Kelly K, Prezant D [2003]. Biomonitoring of chemical exposure among New York City fire fighters responding to the World Trade Center fire and collapse. Environ Health Perspect *111*:1906–1911.

Evans HL [1998]. Mercury. In: Rom WN, editor. Environmental and occupational medicine. 3rd ed. Philadelphia, PA: Lippincott-Raven, pp. 997–1003.

Geomatrix Consultants [2006]. Proposition 65 assessment for antimony trioxide in flame retardant fabrics. Folsom, CA: Geomatrix Consultants, Inc. Project No. 10871.001. Unpublished.

Goldfrank L, Flomenbaum N, Lewin N, Howland MA, Hoffman R, Nelson L [2006]. Goldfrank's toxicologic emergencies. 8th ed. New York, NY: McGraw-Hill Professional, pp. 1244–1250 and 1334-1345.

Harkins DK, Susten AS [2003]. Hair analysis: exploring the state of the science. Environ Health Perspect *111*:576–578.

IARC [1989]. Antimony trioxide and antimony trisulfide. Lyon, France: World Health Organization, International Agency for Research on Cancer [http://www.inchem.org/documents/ iarc/vol47/47-11.html]. Date accessed: March 2009.

Jonsson F, Sandborgh-Englund G, Johanson G [1999]. A compartmental model for the kinetics of mercury vapor in humans. Toxicol Appl Pharmacol *1*:161–168.

Kentner M, Leinemann M, Schaller KH, Weltle D, Lehnert G [1995]. External and internal antimony exposure in starter battery production. Int Arch Occup Environ Health *67*:119–123.

Magos L, Clarkson TW [2006]. Overview of the clinical toxicity of mercury. Ann Clin Biochem *43*:257–268.

NFPA [2009]. NFPA 1975: standard on station/work uniforms for emergency services, 2009 Edition. Quincy, MA: National Fire Protection Association.

NIOSH [1988]. Occupational safety and health guideline for antimony and its compounds (as Sb). Cincinnati, OH: U.S. Department of Health and Human Services, Centers for Disease

REFERENCES
(CONTINUED)

Control and Prevention, National Institute for Occupational Safety and Health [http://www.cdc.gov/Niosh/pdfs/0036.pdf]. Date accessed: March 2009.

Roels HA, Boeckx M, Ceulemans E, Lauwerys RR [1991]. Urinary excretion of mercury after occupational exposure to mercury vapour and influence of the chelating agent meso-2,3-dimercaptosuccinic acid (DMSA). Br J Ind Med 48:247–253.

Seidel S, Kreutzer R, Smith D, McNeel S, Gilliss D [2001]. Assessment of commercial laboratories performing hair mineral analysis. JAMA 258:67–72.

Stokinger HE [1981]. The metals: 2. Antimony, Sb. In: Clayton GD, Clayton FE, editors. Patty's industrial hygiene and toxicology, 3rd ed., Vol. IIA. Toxicology. New York, NY: Wiley-Interscience, pp. 1505–1517.

Taylor JK [1987]. Quality assurance of chemical measurements. Chelsea, MI: Lewis Publishers.

Weidinmyer C, Friedly H [2007]. Mercury emission estimates from fires: an initial inventory for the United States. Environ Sci Technol 31:8092–8098.

Winship KA [1987]. Toxicity of antimony and its compounds. Adv Drug React Acute Poison Rev 2:67–90.

Acknowledgments and Availability of Report

The Hazard Evaluations and Technical Assistance Branch (HETAB) of the National Institute for Occupational Safety and Health (NIOSH) conducts field investigations of possible health hazards in the workplace. These investigations are conducted under the authority of Section 20(a)(6) of the Occupational Safety and Health (OSHA) Act of 1970, 29 U.S.C. 669(a)(6) which authorizes the Secretary of Health and Human Services, following a written request from any employer or authorized representative of employees, to determine whether any substance normally found in the place of employment has potentially toxic effects in such concentrations as used or found. HETAB also provides, upon request, technical and consultative assistance to federal, state, and local agencies; labor; industry; and other groups or individuals to control occupational health hazards and to prevent related trauma and disease.

The findings and conclusions in this report are those of the authors and do not necessarily represent the views of NIOSH. Mention of any company or product does not constitute endorsement by NIOSH. In addition, citations to websites external to NIOSH do not constitute NIOSH endorsement of the sponsoring organizations or their programs or products. Furthermore, NIOSH is not responsible for the content of these websites. All Web addresses referenced in this document were accessible as of the publication date.

This report was prepared by Marie A. de Perio and Srinivas Durgam of HETAB, Division of Surveillance, Hazard Evaluations and Field Studies. Medical field assistance was provided by Judith Eisenberg. Laboratory field assistance was provided by Christine Toennis and John Clark of the Division of Applied Research and Technology at NIOSH. Laboratory analytical support was provided by Kathleen Caldwell of the Inorganic Toxicology Laboratory at the National Center for Environmental Health at CDC. Field assistance and health communication assistance were provided by Stefanie Evans. Editorial assistance was provided by Nicholas Lawryk. Desktop publishing was performed by Robin Smith.

Copies of this report have been sent to employee and management representatives at Boca Raton Fire Rescue Services and Tamarac Fire Rescue, the Florida Department of Health, and the OSHA Regional Office. This report is not copyrighted and may be freely reproduced. The report may be viewed and printed from www.cdc.gov/niosh/hhe. Copies may be purchased from the National Technical Information Service at 5825 Port Royal Road, Springfield, Virginia 22161.

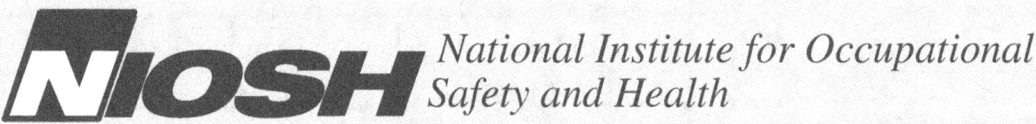

National Institute for Occupational Safety and Health

Delivering on the Nation's promise: Safety and health at work for all people through research and prevention.

To receive NIOSH documents or information about occupational safety and health topics, contact NIOSH at:

1-800-CDC-INFO (1-800-232-4636)

TTY: 1-888-232-6348

E-mail: cdcinfo@cdc.gov

or visit the NIOSH web site at: **www.cdc.gov/niosh.**

For a monthly update on news at NIOSH, subscribe to NIOSH eNews by visiting **www.cdc.gov/niosh/eNews.**

SAFER • HEALTHIER • PEOPLE™

www.ingramcontent.com/pod-product-compliance
Lightning Source LLC
Chambersburg PA
CBHW080941290526
45795CB00007BA/2850